MW01291491

# HEART TUNE-UP JOURNAL AND TRACKER
## 30 Days of Tracking Your Progress In Hindering Heart Disease

ISBN-13: 978-1507849705
ISBN-10: 1507849702

# Free Gift for You

To get your free copy of

"How to Stay Motivated
and Lose Weight"

visit

www.staymotivatedclub.com/tuneup

# MEASURING YOUR SUCCESS

## Weight Loss Chart

| | Weight | Loss |
|---|---|---|
| Week 1 | | |
| Week 2 | | |
| Week 3 | | |
| Week 4 | | |
| Week 5 | | |
| Week 6 | | |
| Week 7 | | |
| Week 8 | | |
| Week 9 | | |
| Week 10 | | |
| Total Loss | | |

## Body Measurements Chart

| Measurement | Week 1 | Week 3 | Week 5 | Week 7 | Week 9 | Inches Lost |
|---|---|---|---|---|---|---|
| Bust | | | | | | |
| Chest | | | | | | |
| Waist | | | | | | |
| Hips | | | | | | |
| Thigh | | | | | | |
| Calves | | | | | | |
| Upper arm | | | | | | |
| Forearm | | | | | | |

# BEFORE PICTURE

**MY WEIGHT**_____

**WHAT I'M THINKING/HOW I FEEL:** _____

_____

_____

_____

_____

_____

_____

# RULES TO FOLLOW

_____

_____

_____

_____

_____

_____

_____

_____

_____

_____

_____

_____

_____

_____

_____

_____

_____

# RULES TO FOLLOW

_____

_____

_____

_____

_____

_____

_____

_____

_____

_____

_____

_____

_____

_____

_____

_____

# TEST RESULTS

| TEST | START | END |
|------|-------|-----|
|      |       |     |
|      |       |     |
|      |       |     |
|      |       |     |
|      |       |     |
|      |       |     |
|      |       |     |
|      |       |     |
|      |       |     |
|      |       |     |
|      |       |     |
|      |       |     |
|      |       |     |
|      |       |     |
|      |       |     |
|      |       |     |
|      |       |     |
|      |       |     |
|      |       |     |
|      |       |     |
|      |       |     |

# TEST RESULTS

| TEST | START | END |
|------|-------|-----|
|      |       |     |
|      |       |     |
|      |       |     |
|      |       |     |
|      |       |     |
|      |       |     |
|      |       |     |
|      |       |     |
|      |       |     |
|      |       |     |
|      |       |     |
|      |       |     |
|      |       |     |
|      |       |     |
|      |       |     |
|      |       |     |
|      |       |     |
|      |       |     |
|      |       |     |
|      |       |     |
|      |       |     |
|      |       |     |
|      |       |     |

# WEEKLY MEAL PLANNER
## Week of _____

|  | BREAKFAST | LUNCH | DINNER | SNACKS |
|---|---|---|---|---|
| **MON** | | | | |
| **TUE** | | | | |
| **WED** | | | | |
| **THU** | | | | |
| **FRI** | | | | |
| **SAT** | | | | |
| **SUN** | | | | |

# DAY 1 – Date_____

## SUPPLEMENTS:  ☐

| | 🕐 | FOOD ITEM | TOTAL FIBER GRAMS |
|---|---|---|---|
| **MEAL 1** | | | |
| | | | |
| | | | |
| **SNACK** | | | |
| **MEAL 2** | | | |
| | | | |
| | | | |
| | | | |
| **SNACK** | | | |
| **MEAL 3** | | | |
| | | | |
| | | | |
| | | | |
| | | **TOTAL** | |

**WATER** 🥛  🥛  🥛  🥛  🥛  🥛  🥛  🥛

## WORKOUTS

| Type | Duration |
|---|---|
| | |
| | |

## NOTES

_____
_____
_____

# DAY 2 – Date_____

## SUPPLEMENTS: ☐

| | 🕐 | FOOD ITEM | TOTAL FIBER GRAMS |
|---|---|---|---|
| **MEAL 1** | | | |
| | | | |
| | | | |
| **SNACK** | | | |
| **MEAL 2** | | | |
| | | | |
| | | | |
| | | | |
| **SNACK** | | | |
| **MEAL 3** | | | |
| | | | |
| | | | |
| | | | |
| | | | |
| | | TOTAL | |

**WATER** ⛾ ⛾ ⛾ ⛾ ⛾ ⛾ ⛾ ⛾

## WORKOUTS

| Type | Duration |
|---|---|
| | |
| | |

## NOTES

_____
_____
_____

## DAY 3 – Date_____

SUPPLEMENTS:  ☐

| | 🕐 | FOOD ITEM | TOTAL FIBER GRAMS |
|---|---|---|---|
| MEAL 1 | | | |
| | | | |
| | | | |
| SNACK | | | |
| MEAL 2 | | | |
| | | | |
| | | | |
| | | | |
| SNACK | | | |
| MEAL 3 | | | |
| | | | |
| | | | |
| | | | |
| | | TOTAL | |

**WATER** 🥛  🥛  🥛  🥛  🥛  🥛  🥛  🥛

### WORKOUTS

| Type | Duration |
|---|---|
| | |
| | |

### NOTES

_____
_____
_____

# DAY 4 – Date_____

SUPPLEMENTS: ☐

| | 🕐 | FOOD ITEM | TOTAL FIBER GRAMS |
|---|---|---|---|
| MEAL 1 | | | |
| | | | |
| | | | |
| SNACK | | | |
| MEAL 2 | | | |
| | | | |
| | | | |
| | | | |
| SNACK | | | |
| MEAL 3 | | | |
| | | | |
| | | | |
| | | | |
| | | TOTAL | |

WATER ☐ ☐ ☐ ☐ ☐ ☐ ☐ ☐

## WORKOUTS

| Type | Duration |
|---|---|
| | |
| | |

## NOTES

_____
_____
_____

# DAY 5 – Date_____

## SUPPLEMENTS: ☐

| | 🕐 | FOOD ITEM | TOTAL FIBER GRAMS |
|---|---|---|---|
| MEAL 1 | | | |
| | | | |
| | | | |
| SNACK | | | |
| MEAL 2 | | | |
| | | | |
| | | | |
| | | | |
| SNACK | | | |
| MEAL 3 | | | |
| | | | |
| | | | |
| | | | |
| | | TOTAL | |

**WATER** 🥛　🥛　🥛　🥛　🥛　🥛　🥛　🥛

## WORKOUTS

| Type | Duration |
|---|---|
| | |
| | |

## NOTES

_____
_____
_____

14

# DAY 6 – Date_____

## SUPPLEMENTS: ☐

| | 🕐 | FOOD ITEM | TOTAL FIBER GRAMS |
|---|---|---|---|
| **MEAL 1** | | | |
| | | | |
| | | | |
| **SNACK** | | | |
| **MEAL 2** | | | |
| | | | |
| | | | |
| | | | |
| **SNACK** | | | |
| **MEAL 3** | | | |
| | | | |
| | | | |
| | | | |
| | | | |
| | | TOTAL | |

**WATER** ▢ ▢ ▢ ▢ ▢ ▢ ▢ ▢

## WORKOUTS

| Type | Duration |
|---|---|
| | |
| | |

## NOTES

_____
_____
_____

## DAY 7 – Date_____

SUPPLEMENTS: ☐

| | 🕐 | FOOD ITEM | TOTAL FIBER GRAMS |
|---|---|---|---|
| MEAL 1 | | | |
| | | | |
| | | | |
| SNACK | | | |
| MEAL 2 | | | |
| | | | |
| | | | |
| | | | |
| SNACK | | | |
| MEAL 3 | | | |
| | | | |
| | | | |
| | | | |
| | | TOTAL | |

WATER ☐  ☐  ☐  ☐  ☐  ☐  ☐  ☐

### WORKOUTS

| Type | Duration |
|---|---|
| | |
| | |

### NOTES

_____
_____
_____

# WEEKLY MEAL PLANNER
## Week of _____

|  | BREAKFAST | LUNCH | DINNER | SNACKS |
|---|---|---|---|---|
| **MON** |  |  |  |  |
| **TUE** |  |  |  |  |
| **WED** |  |  |  |  |
| **THU** |  |  |  |  |
| **FRI** |  |  |  |  |
| **SAT** |  |  |  |  |
| **SUN** |  |  |  |  |

# DAY 8 – Date_____

## SUPPLEMENTS: ☐

| | 🕐 | FOOD ITEM | TOTAL FIBER GRAMS |
|---|---|---|---|
| **MEAL 1** | | | |
| | | | |
| | | | |
| **SNACK** | | | |
| **MEAL 2** | | | |
| | | | |
| | | | |
| | | | |
| **SNACK** | | | |
| **MEAL 3** | | | |
| | | | |
| | | | |
| | | | |
| | | TOTAL | |

**WATER** ⬜ ⬜ ⬜ ⬜ ⬜ ⬜ ⬜ ⬜

## WORKOUTS

| Type | Duration |
|---|---|
| | |
| | |

## NOTES

_____
_____
_____

18

## DAY 9 – Date_____

| | 🕐 | FOOD ITEM | TOTAL FIBER GRAMS |
|---|---|---|---|
| **MEAL 1** | | | |
| | | | |
| | | | |
| **SNACK** | | | |
| **MEAL 2** | | | |
| | | | |
| | | | |
| | | | |
| **SNACK** | | | |
| **MEAL 3** | | | |
| | | | |
| | | | |
| | | | |
| | | **TOTAL** | |

**WATER** ▽  ▽  ▽  ▽  ▽  ▽  ▽  ▽

### WORKOUTS

| Type | Duration |
|---|---|
| | |
| | |

### NOTES

_____
_____
_____

# DAY 10 – Date_____

## SUPPLEMENTS: ☐

| | 🕐 | FOOD ITEM | TOTAL FIBER GRAMS |
|---|---|---|---|
| **MEAL 1** | | | |
| | | | |
| | | | |
| **SNACK** | | | |
| **MEAL 2** | | | |
| | | | |
| | | | |
| **SNACK** | | | |
| **MEAL 3** | | | |
| | | | |
| | | | |
| | | | |
| | | **TOTAL** | |

**WATER** 🥛 🥛 🥛 🥛 🥛 🥛 🥛 🥛

## WORKOUTS

| Type | Duration |
|---|---|
| | |
| | |

## NOTES

_____
_____
_____

## DAY 11 – Date_____

SUPPLEMENTS:  ☐

| | 🕐 | FOOD ITEM | TOTAL FIBER GRAMS |
|---|---|---|---|
| MEAL 1 | | | |
| | | | |
| | | | |
| SNACK | | | |
| MEAL 2 | | | |
| | | | |
| | | | |
| | | | |
| SNACK | | | |
| MEAL 3 | | | |
| | | | |
| | | | |
| | | | |
| | | TOTAL | |

WATER ☐  ☐  ☐  ☐  ☐  ☐  ☐  ☐

### WORKOUTS

| Type | Duration |
|---|---|
| | |
| | |

### NOTES

_____
_____
_____

# DAY 12 – Date_____

## SUPPLEMENTS: ☐

| | 🕐 | FOOD ITEM | TOTAL FIBER GRAMS |
|---|---|---|---|
| **MEAL 1** | | | |
| | | | |
| | | | |
| **SNACK** | | | |
| **MEAL 2** | | | |
| | | | |
| | | | |
| | | | |
| **SNACK** | | | |
| **MEAL 3** | | | |
| | | | |
| | | | |
| | | | |
| | | TOTAL | |

**WATER** ☐ ☐ ☐ ☐ ☐ ☐ ☐ ☐

## WORKOUTS

| Type | Duration |
|---|---|
| | |
| | |

## NOTES

_____
_____
_____

## DAY 13 – Date_____

SUPPLEMENTS: ☐

| | 🕐 | FOOD ITEM | TOTAL FIBER GRAMS |
|---|---|---|---|
| **MEAL 1** | | | |
| | | | |
| | | | |
| **SNACK** | | | |
| **MEAL 2** | | | |
| | | | |
| | | | |
| | | | |
| **SNACK** | | | |
| **MEAL 3** | | | |
| | | | |
| | | | |
| | | | |
| | | **TOTAL** | |

**WATER** ☐  ☐  ☐  ☐  ☐  ☐  ☐  ☐

### WORKOUTS

| Type | Duration |
|---|---|
| | |
| | |

### NOTES

_____
_____
_____

# DAY 14 – Date_____

| | 🕐 | FOOD ITEM | TOTAL FIBER GRAMS |
|---|---|---|---|
| MEAL 1 | | | |
| | | | |
| | | | |
| SNACK | | | |
| MEAL 2 | | | |
| | | | |
| | | | |
| | | | |
| SNACK | | | |
| MEAL 3 | | | |
| | | | |
| | | | |
| | | | |
| | | TOTAL | |

**WATER** ▽  ▽  ▽  ▽  ▽  ▽  ▽  ▽

## WORKOUTS

| Type | Duration |
|---|---|
| | |
| | |

## NOTES

# WEEKLY MEAL PLANNER
## Week of _____

|  | BREAKFAST | LUNCH | DINNER | SNACKS |
|---|---|---|---|---|
| **MON** | | | | |
| **TUE** | | | | |
| **WED** | | | | |
| **THU** | | | | |
| **FRI** | | | | |
| **SAT** | | | | |
| **SUN** | | | | |

# DAY 15 – Date_____

## SUPPLEMENTS: ☐

| | 🕐 | FOOD ITEM | TOTAL FIBER GRAMS |
|---|---|---|---|
| **MEAL 1** | | | |
| | | | |
| | | | |
| **SNACK** | | | |
| **MEAL 2** | | | |
| | | | |
| | | | |
| | | | |
| **SNACK** | | | |
| **MEAL 3** | | | |
| | | | |
| | | | |
| | | | |
| | | TOTAL | |

**WATER** 🥛 🥛 🥛 🥛 🥛 🥛 🥛 🥛

## WORKOUTS

| Type | Duration |
|---|---|
| | |
| | |

## NOTES

_____
_____
_____

# DAY 16 – Date_____

## SUPPLEMENTS: ☐

| | 🕐 | FOOD ITEM | TOTAL FIBER GRAMS |
|---|---|---|---|
| MEAL 1 | | | |
| | | | |
| | | | |
| SNACK | | | |
| MEAL 2 | | | |
| | | | |
| | | | |
| | | | |
| SNACK | | | |
| MEAL 3 | | | |
| | | | |
| | | | |
| | | | |
| | | | |
| | | TOTAL | |

**WATER** ⊔ ⊔ ⊔ ⊔ ⊔ ⊔ ⊔ ⊔

## WORKOUTS

| Type | Duration |
|---|---|
| | |
| | |

## NOTES

_____
_____
_____

## DAY 17 – Date_____

SUPPLEMENTS: ☐

| | 🕐 | FOOD ITEM | TOTAL FIBER GRAMS |
|---|---|---|---|
| MEAL 1 | | | |
| | | | |
| | | | |
| SNACK | | | |
| MEAL 2 | | | |
| | | | |
| | | | |
| | | | |
| SNACK | | | |
| MEAL 3 | | | |
| | | | |
| | | | |
| | | | |
| | | TOTAL | |

WATER ⛾  ⛾  ⛾  ⛾  ⛾  ⛾  ⛾  ⛾

### WORKOUTS

| Type | Duration |
|---|---|
| | |
| | |

### NOTES

28

## DAY 18 – Date_____

SUPPLEMENTS: ☐

| | 🕐 | FOOD ITEM | TOTAL FIBER GRAMS |
|---|---|---|---|
| MEAL 1 | | | |
| | | | |
| | | | |
| SNACK | | | |
| MEAL 2 | | | |
| | | | |
| | | | |
| | | | |
| SNACK | | | |
| MEAL 3 | | | |
| | | | |
| | | | |
| | | | |
| | | TOTAL | |

WATER ☐  ☐  ☐  ☐  ☐  ☐  ☐  ☐

### WORKOUTS

| Type | Duration |
|---|---|
| | |
| | |

### NOTES

29

## DAY 19 – Date_____

| | 🕐 | FOOD ITEM | TOTAL FIBER GRAMS |
|---|---|---|---|
| MEAL 1 | | | |
| | | | |
| | | | |
| SNACK | | | |
| MEAL 2 | | | |
| | | | |
| | | | |
| | | | |
| SNACK | | | |
| MEAL 3 | | | |
| | | | |
| | | | |
| | | | |
| | | TOTAL | |

**WATER** 🥛  🥛  🥛  🥛  🥛  🥛  🥛  🥛

### WORKOUTS

| Type | Duration |
|---|---|
| | |
| | |

### NOTES

_____

_____

_____

# DAY 20 – Date_____

## SUPPLEMENTS: ☐

| | 🕐 | FOOD ITEM | TOTAL FIBER GRAMS |
|---|---|---|---|
| **MEAL 1** | | | |
| | | | |
| | | | |
| **SNACK** | | | |
| **MEAL 2** | | | |
| | | | |
| | | | |
| | | | |
| **SNACK** | | | |
| **MEAL 3** | | | |
| | | | |
| | | | |
| | | | |
| | | | |
| | | TOTAL | |

**WATER** ⊔  ⊔  ⊔  ⊔  ⊔  ⊔  ⊔  ⊔

## WORKOUTS

| Type | Duration |
|---|---|
| | |
| | |

## NOTES

_____
_____
_____

# DAY 21 – Date_____

SUPPLEMENTS: ☐

|  | 🕐 | FOOD ITEM | TOTAL FIBER GRAMS |
|---|---|---|---|
| MEAL 1 |  |  |  |
|  |  |  |  |
|  |  |  |  |
| SNACK |  |  |  |
| MEAL 2 |  |  |  |
|  |  |  |  |
|  |  |  |  |
|  |  |  |  |
| SNACK |  |  |  |
| MEAL 3 |  |  |  |
|  |  |  |  |
|  |  |  |  |
|  |  |  |  |
|  |  | TOTAL |  |

WATER ⊔  ⊔  ⊔  ⊔  ⊔  ⊔  ⊔  ⊔

## WORKOUTS

| Type | Duration |
|---|---|
|  |  |
|  |  |

## NOTES

# WEEKLY MEAL PLANNER
## Week of _____

| | BREAKFAST | LUNCH | DINNER | SNACKS |
|---|---|---|---|---|
| MON | | | | |
| TUE | | | | |
| WED | | | | |
| THU | | | | |
| FRI | | | | |
| SAT | | | | |
| SUN | | | | |

## DAY 22 – Date_____

SUPPLEMENTS: ☐

| | 🕐 | FOOD ITEM | TOTAL FIBER GRAMS |
|---|---|---|---|
| MEAL 1 | | | |
| | | | |
| | | | |
| SNACK | | | |
| MEAL 2 | | | |
| | | | |
| | | | |
| | | | |
| SNACK | | | |
| MEAL 3 | | | |
| | | | |
| | | | |
| | | | |
| | | TOTAL | |

WATER 🥛  🥛  🥛  🥛  🥛  🥛  🥛  🥛

### WORKOUTS

| Type | Duration |
|---|---|
| | |
| | |

### NOTES

## DAY 23 – Date_____

| | 🕐 | FOOD ITEM | TOTAL FIBER GRAMS |
|---|---|---|---|
| MEAL 1 | | | |
| | | | |
| | | | |
| SNACK | | | |
| MEAL 2 | | | |
| | | | |
| | | | |
| | | | |
| SNACK | | | |
| MEAL 3 | | | |
| | | | |
| | | | |
| | | | |
| | | | |
| | | TOTAL | |

**WATER** ☐ ☐ ☐ ☐ ☐ ☐ ☐ ☐

### WORKOUTS

| Type | Duration |
|---|---|
| | |
| | |

### NOTES

_____
_____
_____

# DAY 24 – Date_____

| | 🕐 | FOOD ITEM | TOTAL FIBER GRAMS |
|---|---|---|---|
| MEAL 1 | | | |
| | | | |
| | | | |
| SNACK | | | |
| MEAL 2 | | | |
| | | | |
| | | | |
| | | | |
| SNACK | | | |
| MEAL 3 | | | |
| | | | |
| | | | |
| | | | |
| | | TOTAL | |

**WATER** ☐  ☐  ☐  ☐  ☐  ☐  ☐  ☐

## WORKOUTS

| Type | Duration |
|---|---|
| | |
| | |

## NOTES

_____
_____
_____

# DAY 25 – Date_____

## SUPPLEMENTS:  ☐

| | 🕐 | FOOD ITEM | TOTAL FIBER GRAMS |
|---|---|---|---|
| **MEAL 1** | | | |
| | | | |
| | | | |
| **SNACK** | | | |
| **MEAL 2** | | | |
| | | | |
| | | | |
| | | | |
| **SNACK** | | | |
| **MEAL 3** | | | |
| | | | |
| | | | |
| | | | |
| | | TOTAL | |

**WATER** ▭  ▭  ▭  ▭  ▭  ▭  ▭  ▭

## WORKOUTS

| Type | Duration |
|---|---|
| | |
| | |

## NOTES

_____
_____
_____

# DAY 26 – Date_____

SUPPLEMENTS: ☐

| | 🕐 | FOOD ITEM | TOTAL FIBER GRAMS |
|---|---|---|---|
| MEAL 1 | | | |
| | | | |
| | | | |
| SNACK | | | |
| MEAL 2 | | | |
| | | | |
| | | | |
| SNACK | | | |
| MEAL 3 | | | |
| | | | |
| | | | |
| | | | |
| | | TOTAL | |

WATER ☐  ☐  ☐  ☐  ☐  ☐  ☐  ☐

## WORKOUTS

| Type | Duration |
|---|---|
| | |
| | |

## NOTES

# DAY 27 – Date_____

| | 🕐 | FOOD ITEM | TOTAL FIBER GRAMS |
|---|---|---|---|
| MEAL 1 | | | |
| | | | |
| | | | |
| SNACK | | | |
| MEAL 2 | | | |
| | | | |
| | | | |
| | | | |
| SNACK | | | |
| MEAL 3 | | | |
| | | | |
| | | | |
| | | | |
| | | TOTAL | |

**WATER** ☐  ☐  ☐  ☐  ☐  ☐  ☐  ☐

## WORKOUTS

| Type | Duration |
|---|---|
| | |
| | |

## NOTES

_____
_____
_____

## DAY 28 – Date_____

SUPPLEMENTS: ☐

| | 🕐 | FOOD ITEM | TOTAL FIBER GRAMS |
|---|---|---|---|
| **MEAL 1** | | | |
| | | | |
| | | | |
| **SNACK** | | | |
| **MEAL 2** | | | |
| | | | |
| | | | |
| | | | |
| **SNACK** | | | |
| **MEAL 3** | | | |
| | | | |
| | | | |
| | | | |
| | | TOTAL | |

**WATER** 🥛 🥛 🥛 🥛 🥛 🥛 🥛 🥛

### WORKOUTS

| Type | Duration |
|---|---|
| | |
| | |

### NOTES

_____
_____
_____

# WEEKLY MEAL PLANNER
## Week of _____

| | BREAKFAST | LUNCH | DINNER | SNACKS |
|---|---|---|---|---|
| **MON** | | | | |
| **TUE** | | | | |
| **WED** | | | | |
| **THU** | | | | |
| **FRI** | | | | |
| **SAT** | | | | |
| **SUN** | | | | |

# DAY 29 – Date_____

SUPPLEMENTS: ☐

| | 🕐 | FOOD ITEM | TOTAL FIBER GRAMS |
|---|---|---|---|
| MEAL 1 | | | |
| | | | |
| | | | |
| SNACK | | | |
| MEAL 2 | | | |
| | | | |
| | | | |
| | | | |
| SNACK | | | |
| MEAL 3 | | | |
| | | | |
| | | | |
| | | | |
| | | TOTAL | |

WATER ☐  ☐  ☐  ☐  ☐  ☐  ☐  ☐

## WORKOUTS

| Type | Duration |
|---|---|
| | |
| | |

## NOTES

_____
_____
_____

# DAY 30 – Date_____

| | 🕐 | FOOD ITEM | TOTAL FIBER GRAMS |
|---|---|---|---|
| MEAL 1 | | | |
| | | | |
| | | | |
| SNACK | | | |
| MEAL 2 | | | |
| | | | |
| | | | |
| | | | |
| SNACK | | | |
| MEAL 3 | | | |
| | | | |
| | | | |
| | | | |
| | | TOTAL | |

WATER ⬛ ⬛ ⬛ ⬛ ⬛ ⬛ ⬛ ⬛

## WORKOUTS

| Type | Duration |
|---|---|
| | |
| | |

## NOTES

_____
_____
_____

# AFTER PICTURE

**MY WEIGHT**_____

**WHAT I'M THINKING/HOW I FEEL:** _____

_____

_____

_____

_____

_____

_____

# FAVORITE RECIPES

**Recipe Name:** _____
*Serves:_____*

Oven Temp_____Prep Time_____Cook Time _____

**Ingredients:**

_____        _____

_____        _____

_____        _____

_____        _____

**Preparation Directions:**

_____
_____
_____
_____
_____

**Cooking Directions:**

_____
_____
_____
_____
_____

**Notes:**

_____
_____
_____
_____
_____

# FAVORITE RECIPES

**Recipe Name:** _____
*Serves:*_____

Oven Temp_____Prep Time_____Cook Time _____

**Ingredients:**

_____        _____

_____        _____

_____        _____

_____        _____

**Preparation Directions:**

_____

_____

_____

_____

_____

**Cooking Directions:**

_____

_____

_____

_____

_____

**Notes:**

_____

_____

_____

_____

_____

# FAVORITE RECIPES

**Recipe Name:** _____

*Serves:_____*

Oven Temp_____Prep Time_____Cook Time _____

**Ingredients:**

_____     _____

_____     _____

_____     _____

_____     _____

**Preparation Directions:**

_____

_____

_____

_____

_____

**Cooking Directions:**

_____

_____

_____

_____

_____

**Notes:**

_____

_____

_____

_____

_____

# FAVORITE RECIPES

**Recipe Name:** _____
*Serves:*_____

Oven Temp_____Prep Time_____Cook Time _____

**Ingredients:**

_____     _____

_____     _____

_____     _____

_____     _____

**Preparation Directions:**

_____
_____
_____
_____
_____

**Cooking Directions:**

_____
_____
_____
_____
_____

**Notes:**

_____
_____
_____
_____
_____

# FAVORITE RECIPES

**Recipe Name:** _____
*Serves:_____*

Oven Temp_____Prep Time_____Cook Time _____

**Ingredients:**

_____     _____

_____     _____

_____     _____

_____     _____

**Preparation Directions:**

_____
_____
_____
_____
_____

**Cooking Directions:**

_____
_____
_____
_____
_____

**Notes:**

_____
_____
_____
_____
_____

# FAVORITE RECIPES

**Recipe Name:** _____
*Serves:_____*

Oven Temp_____Prep Time_____Cook Time _____

## Ingredients:

_____          _____

_____          _____

_____          _____

_____          _____

## Preparation Directions:

_____

_____

_____

_____

_____

## Cooking Directions:

_____

_____

_____

_____

_____

## Notes:

_____

_____

_____

_____

_____

# FAVORITE RECIPES

**Recipe Name:** _____
*Serves:*_____

Oven Temp_____Prep Time_____Cook Time _____

**Ingredients:**

_____          _____

_____          _____

_____          _____

_____          _____

**Preparation Directions:**

_____
_____
_____
_____
_____

**Cooking Directions:**

_____
_____
_____
_____
_____

**Notes:**

_____
_____
_____
_____
_____

# FAVORITE RECIPES

**Recipe Name:** _____
*Serves:* _____

Oven Temp_____Prep Time_____Cook Time _____

**Ingredients:**

_____          _____

_____          _____

_____          _____

_____          _____

**Preparation Directions:**

_____
_____
_____
_____
_____

**Cooking Directions:**

_____
_____
_____
_____
_____

**Notes:**

_____
_____
_____
_____
_____

# NOTES

# NOTES

# NOTES

# NOTES

# SHOPPING LIST

# SHOPPING LIST

_____   _____

_____   _____

_____   _____

_____   _____

_____   _____

_____   _____

_____   _____

_____   _____

_____   _____

_____   _____

_____   _____

_____   _____

_____   _____

# SHOPPING LIST

_____    _____

_____    _____

_____    _____

_____    _____

_____    _____

_____    _____

_____    _____

_____    _____

_____    _____

_____    _____

_____    _____

_____    _____

_____    _____

40863706R00035

Made in the USA
San Bernardino, CA
30 October 2016